SHARED GOVERNANCE THAT WORKS

GEN GUANCI
MARKY MEDEIROS

ISBN 13: 978-0-9621520-3-0

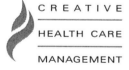

Creative Health Care Management, Inc.
6200 Baker Rd., Suite 200
Minneapolis, Minnesota 55346-1923

www.chcm.com
chcm@chcm.com

800.728.7766 or 952.854.9015

CONTENTS

DEAR **READER**

The Value of Time Spent with You

This book is based on a workshop we've delivered many times throughout the country and on our extensive experience with shared governance in health care organizations. Because demand has been high for our shared governance workshops, we wanted to find a way to help even more people have a successful shared governance experience.

Our solution is this book.

We have compiled the essentials of effective shared governance into a book that can help guide anyone using shared governance for any reason in any setting. Whether you're embarking on a Magnet® or Pathways to Excellence® journey,[1] implementing Relationship-Based Care™, or simply following the expected leadership model in your organization, this book will prepare you to design, implement, and nurture a thriving shared governance structure.

We have learned a lot in the time we've spent with people like you—people who care enough about their organizations to do what it takes to make those organizations better—and we are continually inspired by your intelligence, ingenuity, integrity, and commitment.

---

1. MAGNET®, Magnet Recognition Program®, ANCC®, Magnet®, the Magnet Journey®, and Pathways to Excellence® are registered trademarks of the American Nurses Credentialing Center. The products and services of Creative Health Care Management are neither sponsored nor endorsed by ANCC.

Our wish for you as you read, reflect, discuss, and apply what you learn about shared governance is that you gain enough clarity about the structures and processes involved to move into it with confidence.

As you can guess by the size of this book (and the fact that we didn't name it *Everything You've Ever Wanted to Know About Shared Governance but were Afraid to Ask*), what you're holding is an introduction to shared governance rather than a comprehensive guide. In this book we have provided just the right amount of highly applicable information to help new councils get started and established councils become more effective.

As you move forward, we want you to remember that there is no one-size-fits-all version of shared governance. It will look different in your organization from how it looks in any other. In fact, it may even look a little different in every department in your organization. This book provides you with principles and guidelines, some of which you will follow exactly, and some of which you will customize. You'll choose a model of governance (as described in Chapter Two). The model will evolve over time, and you may even decide to use a completely different model at some point. These changes don't mean you didn't get it right the first time. Because the mission of your organization is always your North Star, you may need to make some changes now and then in order to make sure you're always pointed toward what *you* define as excellence.

We also want you to know this: You were in our hearts and minds as we wrote this book. It is our sincerest wish that you feel supported by what you learn and empowered to make a positive difference in your organization.

To infinity and beyond,

Gen & Marky

CHAPTER **ONE**
Overview of Shared Governance

In the late 1970s and early '80s, health care organizations began practicing a new model of management called *participatory management*. In the participatory management model, staff members participated in some decision making, but leaders retained control of the majority of decisions. As time went by, if trust was established between leaders and staff members, participatory management often morphed into what we now recognize as a shared governance model. The participatory management model of leadership was an important step in the evolution of the shared governance we know today.

Tim Porter-O'Grady, a pioneer in shared governance, defines it as "a structural model through which nurses can express and manage their practice with a higher level of professional autonomy."[2] In addition, Porter-O'Grady considers shared governance to be an organizational framework that enables sustainable, accountability-based decisions. Shared governance is a partnership among all who provide service or support within a health care system.

---

2.   Porter-O'Grady (2003), p.251

Robert Hess, another early leader in the shared governance world, stated in 2004 that shared governance can be elusive, and its structures and processes are different in every organization; he compared the implementation of a shared governance model to pinning Jell-O to a wall. Over time, shared governance has evolved to be less elusive and more readily understood and operationalized. Today, shared governance is used as a leadership and management model and is an everyday practice for many organizations. It helps align the day-to-day practice of a department or unit and to increase ownership in both small and large-scale projects such as the implementation of Relationship-Based Care™ or the journey to excellence. In a journey to excellence, shared governance addresses the professional practice tenet of control of the work environment.

As the shared governance model matured, it became clear to those who used it that in order to serve its purpose, a shared governance structure must be built on a set of overarching principles. Tim Porter-O'Grady identified four overarching principles of shared governance: partnership, equity, accountability, and ownership.[3] We define these essential principles as follows:

Partnership

Staff members and leaders work together at the unit, department, and organization or system level to improve practice and achieve the best outcomes.

Equity

All people contribute within the scope of their roles as part of the team.

Accountability

Staff members and managers share ownership for the outcomes of work; they answer to colleagues, the organization, and the community they serve.

---

3. Porter-O'Grady (2009)

Ownership
> Participants accept that success is linked to how well they do their individual jobs.

Through operationalizing these principles, organizations began to see their work cultures shift from an *us vs. them* mentality to a culture of *we*.

Porter-O'Grady notes in his Foreword to Swihart & Hess's *Shared Governance: A Practical Approach to Transforming Interprofessional Healthcare*, that only 10% of unit- and department-level decisions should be made by management.[4] While some organizations still oppose shared governance (or confuse it with participatory management), others are moving toward a shared governance culture. Unfortunately, many organizations are pursuing shared governance without adequate knowledge of best practices seen throughout the country.

Bureaucracy and Hierarchy

Health care organizations have traditionally been bureaucratic in nature. Whether we like it or not, hierarchy remains the basic structure of most, if not all, ongoing human systems. Without some hierarchy, in situations in which people are expected to work together, there may not be enough structure for people to be productive.

Merriam-Webster defines *hierarchy* as a body of persons in authority; the classification of a group of people according to ability or to economic, social, or professional standing.[5] You probably know from experience that bureaucracies can be characterized by:

- Complex or indirect communications

---

4. Swihart & Hess (2014)
5. "Hierarchy," *Merriam-Webster Online*

- Workarounds

- A tendency toward excessive documentation

- A tendency toward excessive policies, procedures, and protocols

Organizational Leadership Styles

The larger an organization is, the more complex the structures will be, and the larger the variety of leadership styles can be observed. The continuum shown in Figure 1.1 depicts the range of organizational leadership styles. On the far left is *autocracy*, which connotes an organization in which one person decides everything. On the far right is *self-directed teams,* which connotes an organization in which teams are empowered to decide for themselves, and with each other, without additional supervision, how best to accomplish their work.

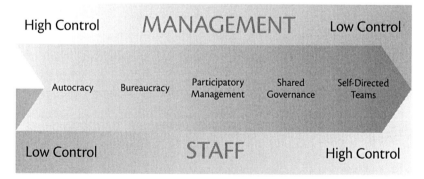

Figure 1.1: Empowerment and Control Continuum[6]

As you can see, the levels of control shift, commensurate with the different organizational structures. While it may sound risky for people in management to cede some measure of control to

6.   Reprinted from Creative Health Care Management (2015)

the staff, a carefully crafted shared governance structure ensures that staff members are equipped to function effectively as they take far greater ownership of their work.

Perhaps you can imagine a time or place within health care when each of the styles depicted in Figure 1.1 would be appropriate.

Autocracy

Autocracy means that one person makes the decisions. For example, during a time of crisis, such as a cardiac arrest, it is in the patient's best interest to have one person in charge and giving directions. This ensures that team members are all moving in the same direction.

Bureaucracy

Bureaucracy is characterized by standardized procedures (rule-following), formal division of responsibility, hierarchy, and impersonal relationships. For example, in order to change an organizational policy, the proposed change must be brought to the leaders responsible for review, revision, and approval.

Participatory Management

Participatory management is characterized by managers or leaders gathering input from the staff, then making the final decisions. For example, a leader asks for staff input on the upcoming work schedule. The leader then takes that input and makes the final schedule decisions, which may or may not reflect all staff input.

Shared Governance

Shared governance is an organizational framework that enables sustainable, accountability-based decisions that are made closest to the point of care.[7] Here's an example of shared governance in action: The practice council is asked to decide what IV pumps to purchase. The leader shares the criteria that the council decision must meet. The council determines which pump(s) meet the criteria and informs leadership. These pumps are purchased.

Self-Directed Teams

Nearly unheard of in health care, a self-directed team comprises people who are fully empowered to do their jobs without supervision. They confer and collaborate with each other as needed, and any individual may step up temporarily to lead a specific project as needed. Self-directed teams may or may not have complete discretion over a budget.

Shared Governance as a Key Expression of Organizational Culture

Organizational culture can be thought of as the collective personality of an organization. Culture is the key to what can and cannot survive in any organization and even in an individual department, unit, or shift. While some intentions about culture can be formalized, organizational culture is ultimately unwritten—and often unspoken—and can vary from department to department, unit to unit, even shift to shift. Culture develops over time and, once established, can remain relatively stable. Furthermore, culture is strongly influenced by leaders.[8]

In order for a shared governance culture to flourish, there are issues and concerns that must be addressed early in development of its structures and processes, and then re-addressed

---

7.   Porter-O'Grady (2003)

8.   Guanci (2015)

frequently. Among these issues is leaders' concern about loss of power and control or feeling that shared governance asks them to abdicate their leadership role. Staff member issues include the concern that shared governance positions them to do their leaders' work with no pay increase or promotion, as well as confusion about their scope of responsibility and authority. In addition to leadership and staff issues, organizational issues most likely to adversely affect the shared governance culture are lack of a sustainment plan and a culture of blame.

Potential Barriers to Shared Governance

Barriers to establishing shared governance can be placed into two groups: 1) limited resources, or 2) lack of specific structural requirements. Limited resources might include limited time, money, and people to participate. Lack of structural requirements could include lack of support from management or the organization itself, lack of trust, lack of competence or confidence among staff members, and lack of a culture in which errors are thought of as opportunities to learn, rather than reasons for shame or punishment.

Benefits of Shared Governance

There is strong support in the literature for the many benefits of a shared governance culture, for the organization as a whole and for units and individuals.[9] Benefits most often cited are higher staff satisfaction and retention and stronger staff ownership of data and outcomes such as patient experience and improved work environment. Staff members participating in shared governance also express appreciation for their increased autonomy and a stronger sense of meaning and purpose in their work.

---

9. Guanci (2005); Guanci (2007); Guanci (2015); Manojlovich (2007); McClure & Hinshaw (2002); Porter-O'Grady (1992); Swihart & Hess (2014)

Shared Governance versus Participatory Management

One challenge facing organizations and leaders implementing shared governance is understanding the difference between participatory management and shared governance. When comparing these two decision-making models, the following five foci must be considered: 1) goals, 2) use of staff input, 3) how decisions are made, 4) leadership style, which includes presence and philosophy, and 5) the level at which decisions are made. The two models approach each of these five foci differently, as summarized in Figure 1.2.

Participatory Management	Shared Governance
Goals	**Goals**
Leaders request input from staff to determine goals; use of input is optional.	Staff are given the responsibility, authority, and accountability to determine what goals to pursue.
Use of staff input	**Use of staff input**
Leader is not required to use staff input.	Staff obtains and incorporates input from colleagues and others.
How decisions are made	**How decisions are made**
Final decision lies with leader, who may accept or reject staff input.	Leaders clearly articulate the guidelines for the decision (e.g., We have $10,000 to spend on ___), and staff are empowered to autonomously make decisions that stay within the guidelines.
Leadership style	**Leadership style**
Hierarchical leader	Servant leader

Participatory Management	Shared Governance
Level at which decisions are made	Level at which decisions are made
Centralized decision making	Decentralized decision making

Figure 1.2: Shared Governance versus Participatory Management[10]

Shared Governance: What It Is, and What It Is Not

Shared governance IS:

- A model that ensures that decisions are made by people working at the point of care

- A leadership development strategy

- A way to identify future positional leaders

- A tenet of professional practice

- A key expression of organizational culture

Shared governance IS NOT:

- The replacement or elimination of positional leadership

- A strategy to support downsizing of leadership

- Self-governance

A vibrant shared governance model leads to improvements in practice and in the patient experience. When shared governance is well-designed and leaders and staff members know how

---

10. Adapted from Guanci (2015)

to participate, "stars are born," as people with great ideas and the energy to enact change emerge.

The remainder of this book will cover the key structures and processes needed for shared governance that works!

"The measure of who we are is what we do with what we have."

~ Vince Lombardi

CHAPTER TWO
Shared Governance Structures

The way you structure shared governance can greatly enhance the success of your endeavor. Consider including a diverse group of people from various units and departments and from different levels in the organization who will decide what your model will look like. This group is often called the steering group, which we will describe more fully in a moment.

Two Models of Shared Governance

The literature features three models of shared governance: the Administrative Model, the Congressional Model, and the Councilor Model.[11] Because the Administrative Model perpetuates a more bureaucratic structure, we will focus in this book only on the two models that lend themselves to a more authentically decentralized decision-making structure.

---

11.   Porter-O'Grady (1992)

The Congressional Model

The Congressional Model, depicted in Figure 2.1, empowers participants to vote on issues as a group. In a congressional model, a congress—a group that addresses organization-wide concerns—is made up of constituents from various departments. The congress ensures that clinical decisions are made at the point of care or service, and it focuses on practice issues that affect multiple areas.

This model has an executive cabinet—often chaired by a clinical staff person—which provides strategic and operational direction and is responsible for improving processes within the shared governance system. Specialty councils in this model include but are not limited to a nursing practice council and a human resources council. Standing committees in a congressional model include education, quality, and practice committees. Standing committees carry out the work of the congress, providing structure for the implementation of practice changes as well as subsequent evaluation of the change.

The staff member who leads the congress is elected and is relieved of anywhere from 50% to 100% of their everyday duties to make space for their shared governance work.

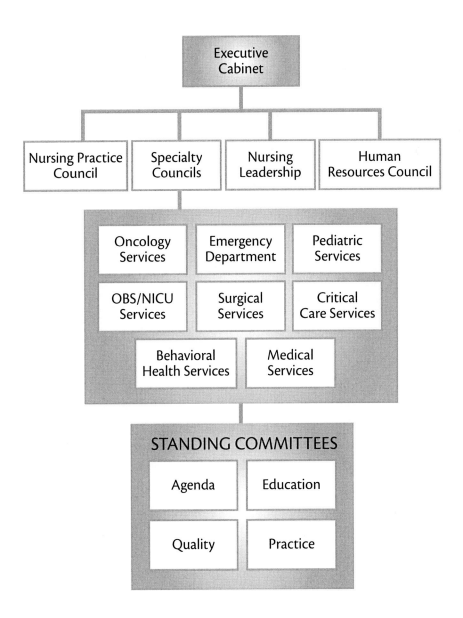

Figure 2.1: The Congressional Model of Shared Governance

The Councilor Model

The most common shared governance decision-making model—and the one we believe to be most supportive of it—is the Councilor Model, shown in Figure 2.2. The Councilor Model is made up of a coordinating council, central councils, and unit-based councils.

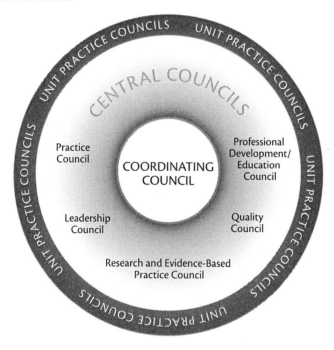

Figure 2.2: The Council Model of Shared Governance

Coordinating Council

The coordinating council is responsible for overseeing the structures and processes that hold the shared governance model together. Members of the coordinating council review the bylaws and charters of each unit practice council, create templates for standardization, and are the go-to group when questions arise as to which council a certain agenda item should belong to. The coordinating council may be made up of chairs from the central councils. This council also receives reports and updates of activities happening in the central councils and often from unit- or department-level councils as well.

Central Councils

Central councils are organizational councils with a specific focus, and they can vary from organization to organization. Small organizations may have fewer councils covering more than one purpose. Often organizations will have these councils and others:

- Practice Council

- Research and Evidence-Based Practice Council

- Quality Council

- Leadership Council

- Professional Development/Education Council

Often the model evolves so that five years after implementation you may add and/or combine councils to refine and/or grow the structure in your organization.

Unit Practice Councils (also referred to as Unit Councils, Unit-Based Councils, Staff Councils, or Unit/Department Service Councils)

Councils can vary in makeup from unit to unit. In some cases, they may represent a department or even a broader service line. In any case, they should be made up mostly of staff members who work at the point of care or service, and should focus on issues involving practice or service, the practice or work environment, performance improvement, and professional development. Unit practice councils are where decisions related to unit- or department-specific practices are made. These unit councils provide a venue for the voices of staff members.

Determining Which Structure is Best for Your Organization

The work of determining the structure of shared governance often lies with a steering group made up of members from throughout the organization. Because this group works to determine what structure will work best within the organization, it's important that it includes members from all levels of the organization and from various divisions, departments, units, and settings. Whenever practical, invite interprofessional partners to take part in the planning and creation phase of nursing councils.

First steps may include examining various models from other organizations, conducting literature searches on shared governance models, and inviting experts in to support the work of creating councils. Think together about what it will take to get started. Think about which councils could start in the first phase, in the second phase, and so on. Consider nursing councils, unit- or department-based councils, and interprofessional councils, each of which will follow overarching council bylaws and may then be further customized as appropriate.

Desired **activities** for the steering group include:

- Group education on shared governance models

- Education and feedback from others in the organization regarding the models

- Education on the decision-making process (consensus) and how it is accomplished

- Education on the first steps of preparation for implementation of the councils

Desired **outcomes** for the steering group include:

- Identification of the shared governance model for the organization

- Implementation of consensus decision-making

- Development of a draft of shared governance bylaws/ guidelines

- Development of implementation requirements such as a membership recruitment strategy

The initial work of the steering group will be completed once the model (councilor or congressional) and number and type of councils is decided. This group should remain in place while the remaining structures and processes are developed, potentially including the development of bylaws and guidelines, a membership recruitment strategy, and the processes by which you will ensure that councils receive the education needed to be successful.

Writing Shared Governance Bylaws for the Organization's Shared Governance System

Bylaws are an important part of a shared governance structure. At a minimum, one set of bylaws outlines the purpose of shared governance, the purpose of each council, and the function of the councils. Bylaws provide the structure the shared governance model works from and guide operations of the councils. The drafting of bylaws is usually done by a group selected by the steering group to coordinate council activities and receive reports from all other councils. In the Councilor Model, this group is sometimes referred to as a coordinating council. The document they create might range from two to several dozen pages long. Generally speaking, brief and meaningful is better than long and involved. It may be helpful to look at other organizations' bylaws before drafting bylaws for your organization. Several excellent samples of shared governance bylaws are available on the internet. When creating bylaws, reflect on and include the following:

Philosophy
What is your organization's philosophy? How might shared governance match or advance your organization's philosophy?

Responsibilities
What will council members, leaders, chairs and co-chairs be responsible for?

Authority
What is the council authorized to decide and do? What is not within the purview of the council to decide or do?

Accountability
Who has accountability for what?

Membership
Who will make up the council? (Think in terms of roles, not individuals' names.)

Decision Making
How will decisions be made? Will the best practice of consensus decision making be the primary methodology?

When the bylaws are finalized, they can be disseminated to all council chairs once the chairs are in place. Bylaws are reviewed annually at the council meetings, and any proposed amendments are forwarded to the coordinating council for consideration. Some unit councils and organizational councils customize council bylaws, charters, or guidelines to specify the purpose, membership, and guiding principles of each council.

Establishing Charters and Guidelines

Each council is responsible for creating its own charter or set of guidelines based on the bylaws of the shared governance model. These documents must never contradict the bylaws established by the coordinating council. A charter can be as brief as two pages but can be longer. The charter states the council's purpose, membership, guiding principles, responsibilities, and goals. Charters and guidelines should be reviewed annually and amended as necessary.

Determining Membership

When discussing the structure of councils, membership is one of the most important things to consider. For organizational councils, make sure to have staff representation from different units and departments, including, whenever possible, interprofessional colleagues. It is a best practice to have councils led by a staff member. Often organizational councils will designate a mentor from the leadership team to coach the staff chairperson.

While membership will look different from council to council, a council generally comprises a chair or chairs and general staff-level membership. This membership could include leaders who are there as observers and/or informal facilitators, interprofessional partners, and ad hoc members. An outside facilitator may also be present. (See page 52 for more on facilitators.) All members must know their roles and responsibilities on the council, as defined in the principles and bylaws.

Members can join councils in a variety of ways. In some organizations there is an election process in which a person runs for the position of member and is elected to be on the council. There may be an election process for the chair and co-chair as well.

More often than not, it is a volunteer process where interested people volunteer to be on the council.

Another membership identification best practice is a nomination process in which all people in a work area are asked the question, "Which co-workers from our unit or department would you choose to make decisions for our unit or department?" The individuals with the most nominations are then invited to join the council.

When members rotate off the council over time, new members may enter through a request for new members (volunteer or nominations process) or may be recruited by a fellow council member. People may also be asked to be on the council because of their expertise in a certain area.

Ensuring Membership Commitment

Membership considerations are not limited to who should be included, but also how many people to include, how they become members, how long the commitment is, and how, when, and why members will rotate off the council. Include in the bylaws a clear statement of the expectations for attendance and the consequences for non-attendance. A common standard for attendance is 75-80% of council meetings before a replacement is considered due to non-attendance. (See Figure 2.3, Commitment to Serve template on page 24.)

Establishing Meeting Times

Include in the bylaws 1) when the council will meet, 2) how long the meetings will be, and 3) how often, and make sure the meeting time is paid protected time. Council members must be able to get away from the unit or department if the meeting is during a work shift or be able to request not to be scheduled on the unit during council meetings. Either way, council members' time at meetings must be protected time and paid time. If this is not the case, it will quickly become clear to all that the organization is not really committed to shared governance.

Determining Responsibilities of Council Chairs and Co-Chairs

As previously stated, councils are led by staff members rather than managers. These chairs and co-chairs are responsible for a variety of tasks.

Planning the Agenda

At the organization level, agenda planning may be handled by the council chair and the mentor on the council. Agenda items may be carried over from one meeting to the next. Items may come up in the meeting that need to go on the agenda for the next meeting. The purpose and goals of the council will determine what is on the agenda. Some councils will have standing agenda items. It is important to periodically assess the value of individual standing items; keep standing items that prove essential over time, and discard any items that take too much time and provide too little value.

Posting Agendas One Week Before Each Meeting

Agendas should be posted or emailed ahead of time, so members can prepare for discussions.

Organizing Speakers for Meetings

A council may determine that it is necessary for someone to present information at the next meeting. The presenters may be members of the council, leaders in the organization, people in the organization whose work is interdependent with the work of the council, or people from outside the organization. The chair is responsible for making sure speakers are invited to attend the meeting. Presenters may include:

- Pharmacists, regarding issues with medications

- Patient experience personnel, regarding patient satisfaction data

- The CNO, regarding the nursing strategic plan

- The unit or department leader, regarding initiatives in the work area that will be communicated to different departments

- Interprofessional colleagues or people from other departments whose partnership must be sought in order to design work that will affect multiple professions or work areas

Other responsibilities of the chairperson or co-chairs include running meetings and following up after them, as described below.

Leading Meetings

The chairperson introduces agenda items, asks questions, provides insight, and generally keeps the meeting going. The council chair may delegate facilitation of group process and/or minute taking to another group member.

Reviewing and Distributing Meeting Minutes

The chairperson is responsible for reviewing the minutes, sending them out to members for approval, and posting them once approved. Posting may be by email to the unit or coordinating council, to an intranet shared governance webpage, to a shared online resource in your organization, or on a unit or department bulletin board. Your councils will determine the process for posting minutes. It is important that the minutes be actively distributed rather than passively posted where people will find them only if they choose to go looking for them.

Following up

There may be follow-up after the meeting, with assignments for others or for the council chair (e.g., literature searches, data gathering). The chair is responsible for assigning this work. The chair does not have to do all the work but coordinates the work to keep people on track.

Decision Making

The form of decision making the councils will use is outlined in the bylaws. Consensus decision making is a best practice in shared governance. The council chair is responsible for ensuring that consensus decision making is happening consistently in the group. Consensus will be discussed in detail in Chapter Three.

Monitoring Attendance

Attendance is a common challenge for councils—especially new shared governance councils. As previously stated, it is important to set guidelines for attendance, and it is up to the council chair (or a designee) to monitor whether or not people are keeping their attendance commitments. If a group member's attendance is unsatisfactory, ask if the person is still committed to the group. If the person is not, find a replacement. The group's charter and bylaws will specify a minimum attendance percentage which should be agreed to by all members (for example, 80%). Consequences should also be outlined for those failing to keep their commitments, and it is the chair's role to administer the consequences.

A best practice to support commitment to attendance is having each council member sign a Commitment to Serve document. This document outlines expectations of council members, including attendance requirements. Figure 2.3 is a sample Commitment to Serve document.

While the list of council chair responsibilities is lengthy, the responsibility can be shared with a co-chair, or support may be provided from a previous chair until the new chair is comfortable with the new responsibilities. Chairing councils is a great way to hone leadership skills and to develop professionally. The chairperson learns how to lead meetings, deal with differing opinions, facilitate consensus decision making, address changes in practice or service that may ensue from council decisions, and conduct follow up after meetings. Organizations with professional advancement programs or clinical ladders often award points for chairing a council.

Shared governance chairs are often looked to when leadership positions open. Whether it be unit-level positions, manager positions, or a chance to advance from participation on a unit council to participation on an organizational council, shared governance chairs are often offered opportunities for advancement.

Commitment to Serve [Template]

(While this example is written for nursing, it can be easily adapted for any council and any area.)

Congratulations on becoming a member of the [organization's name] Shared Governance [council name] Council!

This will be an exciting opportunity for you to represent the nursing department, your unit, and your workgroup as we ensure decision making by those most involved with practice and the care of our patients.

In your role as a [council name] **Council Member**, you will be involved with defining, implementing, and maintaining high standards of nursing clinical practice consistent with national, regional, and community standards, and evaluating services and outcomes within your scope of responsibility.

As a council member you have the following responsibilities:

- Attend at least 80% [or whatever your % requirement is] of the _____ Council meetings. The meetings will be held on [add your day and time structure here].
- Schedule yourself to attend these meetings, with the assistance of your manager/leader as needed.
- Notify the council chair if you are unable to attend a meeting.
- Disseminate council activities and information back to your unit.
- Gather feedback and suggestions from your colleagues to assist in decision making.
- Complete council work and/or assignments within the required timeline.
- Engage in solutions that improve patient care outcomes, patient experiences, and the professional environment.
- Be emotionally present during meetings.

Participation in the professional governance structure for nursing at [organization's name] is an honor and commitment to both your profession and your colleagues. Please recognize that your participation is highly valued and respected by your peers and the Nursing Management Team.

• • •

By virtue of my signature below, I accept my appointment, understand my responsibilities, and intend to serve in my fullest capacity.

_____   _____
Council Member   Date

_____   _____
Name/Credentials/Title   Date

[Note: Some organizations have their CNO, Director of Professional Practice, or Magnet Director as the signer.]

Figure 2.3: Commitment to Serve Template

Ten Ideas to Encourage Council Meeting Attendance

1. Consider time of day/night. Ask council members for input into meeting times.

2. Make meetings interesting. Have a hot topic on the agenda; if people want to hear what is going to happen, they will attend.

3. Keep meetings focused on what is meaningful to the group. Meeting activities should be about the work and the work environment.

4. Make practice changes that are visible and meaningful. Start with small changes, and celebrate what works. Then build to bigger changes.

5. Vary speakers and responsibilities. It's more interesting when new people come to present information, rather than the same person presenting every time.

6. Invite people to come because of their expertise or passion. For example, if the council is discussing patient satisfaction data, have an expert come and talk about the survey questions, graphs, etc.

7. Make sure everyone is heard. There are natural introverts and extroverts. Ask to hear from the people who don't often speak up, and don't let one or two people monopolize the discussions.

8. Communicate decisions and new ideas. Create a newsletter, send out emails of the top five takeaways from meetings, create a communication tree.

9. Provide food and drink. Providing snacks or treats is a great way to get people to come to meetings.

10. Make it fun!

Providing Standardized Council Templates

Develop or adapt a set of templates for councils to use, and have a designated place where shared governance templates and documents are saved and shared. Recommended templates include those for:

- Bylaws

- Agendas

- Meeting minutes

- Annual reports—goals, projects, year-end reports

- Individual council template for that council's specific purpose, focused work, membership, role/responsibilities

Communication in shared governance is essential.

Establishing Structures for Communicating Information

Porter-O'Grady states, "Although every existing tool is used to communicate, there is often poor penetration."[12] In order to address this poor communication penetration, what happens in the meetings needs to be communicated to all stakeholders. For unit practice councils, that means everyone on the unit must know how to find out what happened at the meeting. For central or organizational councils, that means all professionals must know how to find out what happened at the practice council, quality council, and research council meetings.

There must also be a process for non-members to communicate with the councils. How do people who are not on the council

12. Porter-O'Grady (2009), p. 260

bring an issue to the council? Do they discuss the issue with a designated unit representative? Is there a place on the council website to submit questions and concerns?

Finally, a process is also needed for communication between councils. If all central council chairs are members of the coordinating council, communication is simplified. In addition, be sure the minutes of each council are posted in a place where all have access for reviewing purposes. If there is an issue in one council that needs to go to another council, how does that communication take place?

Means of spreading the messages include newsletters, bulletin boards, communication trees, presentations, staff meetings and huddles, and shared online resources.

Articulating Leader and Staff Expectations

Shared governance structures provide opportunities for decision making to be shared by stakeholders who have the most impact on making changes and improving outcomes. Decisions formerly made by leaders are now made by staff members within clearly articulated guidelines. There are new roles for both leaders and staff members that may be uncomfortable at first.

Porter-O'Grady put it this way: "Leadership is no longer managership. The whole role of leader is directed to facilitating the growth of leadership in all roles in the system."[13]

Expectations of Leaders

As the expectations of leaders change in a shared governance environment, fundamental leadership roles emerge. These include:

- Being a resource for clinical staff

---

13. Porter-O'Grady (2009), p. 8

- Inspiring and affirming council work
- Coaching and mentoring council chairs and co-chairs
- Ensuring paid, protected time for council work
- Meeting with the chairs/co-chairs to discuss the work of the council
- Supporting chairs in agenda development
- Providing tools to complete unit projects
- Clearly articulating expectations of councils
- Defining council tasks
- Managing conflict
- Aligning council work with goals
- Fostering civility
- Facilitating open communication
- Modeling confidence and optimism

It's important to remember that the role of leaders in shared governance is just as important as it is in any other decision-making structure. The role simply changes to one of making space for the larger group—particularly the people closest to the work—to determine their own priorities and design their own work processes.

The Leader's Role on the Council

Shared governance is not an outright turning over of the reins to staff to make decisions. There are decisions that require staff members' input, and there are decisions that only leaders have authority to make. Decisions regarding practice, the practice environment, and professional practice belong to staff members. Again, Porter-O'Grady shares insight: "The locus of control in empowered organizations is at the point of service where most of the decisions are made."[14] Leaders have distinct roles in relation to councils. Their work is to set and articulate guidelines for decisions, coach and mentor staff leaders, and foster a culture of accountability. They provide resources and support as needed, establish norms for looking at different points of view, engage members in problem solving, and encourage two-way communication. Above all, leaders must resolve to let things change in the work environment, allowing staff members the freedom to experiment and perhaps to make mistakes.

Expectations of Council Members

Members must be prepared to work hard. There may be assignments that need to be completed outside of council time. Members must be engaged in and committed to the work. The primary focus of unit councils is practice and the practice environment. Members must see the need for change and apply themselves to the task of designing and implementing those changes. They must be willing and able to maintain honesty, openness, realism, and tact. As things unfold, missteps are inevitable. It's important for people to stay positive and keep moving toward the goals of the council. Success can be measured in improved outcomes including patient outcomes, patient satisfaction, and employee satisfaction.

Council work is often different from what staff members are used to doing. Expectations include:

- Bringing issues to the council

- Actively participating in discussions and decisions

---

14. Porter-O'Grady (2009), p. 13

- Completing literature searches on specific topics
- Communicating information from council meetings to colleagues
- Soliciting feedback from others in the unit
- Reviewing materials prior to council meetings
- Serving on ad hoc committees and workgroups
- Attending meetings according to the bylaws and charter of the council

Educating Shared Governance Councils

Implementing shared governance in an organization often presents a new way of doing things, so it's important to address the educational needs that go along with implementation. Determine how to educate people about the shared governance model, including providing a full explanation of the reason for the change. While this book provides information about what shared governance is and how it is accomplished, only people within the organization can help others understand why this new model of decision making is being established. Shared governance both signals and advances a positive cultural shift that promotes a high level of staff member commitment to their work.

In addition to educating members of the councils and others in the organization, chairs and co-chairs of councils need specific education. For chairs, consider providing education three to four times a year on a variety of leadership topics, with the first session addressing how to run a meeting, how to plan an agenda, how to review minutes, leadership skills, how to write goals, and how to communicate effectively.

Understanding Stages of Council Development

Councils are teams (groups of people linked in a common purpose), and teams go through predictable stages of development. A team becomes more than just a collection of people when a strong sense of mutual commitment creates synergy. Cohesive teams take time to build, yet most teams are expected to start functioning efficiently from Day One. This is an unfair expectation; teams need time to build.

Bruce Tuckman, in a paper that has become a classic, described four stages of team building: forming, storming, norming, and performing.[15] Each stage has its own member concerns and role for leadership. Tuckman's terminology, combined with the further scholarship of Dave Francis and Don Young, provides helpful insight into the development and evolution of councils.[16] Figure 2.4 summarizes this evolution in terms of how group members tend to interact and what they can accomplish at each stage.

---

15. Tuckman (1965)
16. Francis & Young (1979)

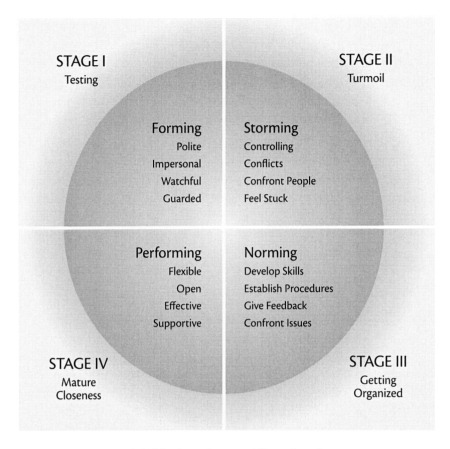

Figure 2.4: The Four Stages of Team Development

Forming

When groups form, they are in the exploratory stage in which first impressions play a significant part. Individuals in this stage experience a variety of emotions, including confusion, anxiety, and excitement. Many will approach the group politely, cautiously, and watchfully, and will be guarded in their interactions. During this stage, it is important to spend time addressing the issue of inclusion. Allowing time for individuals to address their initial concerns around belonging, before jumping into the work of the group, will be time well spent. People will naturally go through some personal inquiry into the ways in which they do or perhaps do not feel they belong in the group. Inquiries can be broad: Why am I here? Do I want to be here? Or they can be deep: Will I be accepted? What price will I pay to belong to this team? During this forming stage, leaders need to share relevant information and provide structure. Encouraging open dialogue helps develop a climate of trust and respect among individuals, the group, and leadership. Taking time for group development, rather than attempting to dive right into the work before trust and camaraderie are established, can be very beneficial for the group's long-term success.

Storming

During this stage, groups often experience various degrees of turmoil. Competition and struggles may arise, often over who will lead, how decisions will be made, and what the balance of control or power will be. This can lead to defensiveness, frustration, feeling stuck, and even anger. Development of informal subgroups is common during this stage. These are groups of people who sit together at the meetings, have sidebar conversations, push the same agenda, and/or do not listen to what others have to say.

As in the forming stage, it's important in the storming stage to allow time for the group to work through issues of inclusion. People will begin to notice when others seem to have control over them or they seem to have control over others. They'll question whose support they have, and they may support some people within the group more than others. They'll notice how much influence they have inside the team versus elsewhere in the world.

Leadership continues to have an important role during the storming stage, including engaging members in group problem solving, establishing norms for looking at different viewpoints, encouraging two-way communication, supporting collaborative team efforts, and exercising patience as the group works through this difficult stage. It is important for staff members and leaders alike to openly discuss the consensus decision-making process during this stage.

Norming

In the norming stage, the group is transitioning into a team and establishing harmony. Trust and respect grow as the group develops cohesiveness, appreciates differences, shares responsibility, and displays interdependent behavior through team problem solving. There may be a renegotiation of roles during this stage, and there is most certainly increased satisfaction. A healthy team is one in which members feel safe in expressing differences of opinion in a respectful way.

Team members address, individually and together, their issues related to inclusion. Over time people notice that they can be successful as a team, and they can then more clearly look at ways to measure their successes.

As the team matures during the norming stage, the leader's role evolves to one of coach and mentor—leading from behind. The leader must establish and maintain a strong communication process with council leads, continue to articulate the guidelines by which decisions must be made, talk openly about issues and concerns, give positive and constructive feedback, encourage team members to manage team process, and, most importantly, support consensus decision making.

Performing

In this stage, the group has become a team working together with open communication, shared goals, and clear outcome expectations. Members have worked out relationships; they manage conflicts and are confident and optimistic. Because they are all pointed toward the same clear goals, their work is focused on the tasks needed to meet team goals and outcomes.

Issues of inclusion do not exist in this stage, since they have been worked out in previous stages. Leadership continues to lead from behind, coaching and guiding council leads without directing them. The most important role for leadership during this stage is to stay out of the way.

One Important Caveat

It is quite common, and should be expected, that a team will return to a prior level of development when there is a change in leadership or even membership. When one person leaves or joins, the team is changed. The team is then forced to work through the beginning stages of forming and storming. Failure to return to the forming and storming phases when new members are added is the most common cause of poor performance of councils. Although it might seem ideal for a high-performing team to continue on its track when new members or leaders rotate in, what an uninterrupted continuation actually indicates is that the new people have not been integrated into the team. This is one reason why meeting attendance is limited to council members and others who have been specifically invited. Everyone on the team has a role, and time should be taken to articulate these roles as councils develop, particularly if membership and/or council leadership changes.

Moving Forward: Essential Questions for Steering and Coordinating Councils to Consider

We suggest reflecting as a group on these important questions. The questions are essential at the start and are worth revisiting as councils begin to take shape.

1. **How many councils will there be at the organizational level?**

   Consider practice councils and leadership councils, as well as councils guiding and measuring research, quality, and more.

2. **How will unit-based councils be configured?**

   Some organizations have unit-based councils for every unit, department, and/or service line. Outpatient departments and clinics could have several councils each or just one, depending on the size of their department.

3. **What other professions would ideally be represented on the councils?**

   Consider members representing pharmacy, occupational and physical therapy, social work, and nutrition services. Remember to invite physician colleagues.

4. **How will the organization be educated about shared governance?**

   Determine how leaders and staff members will be helped to understand the new model and its guiding principles and how chairs of other councils will be educated.

5. **How will strategic planning occur?**

   One of the most effective ways to facilitate all the councils working together as a team is to have a shared governance strategic planning retreat. Strategic planning is a way to share the vision, goals, organizational priorities, and expectations for the coming year. It's a great way to focus on priorities, goals, and outcomes.

6. **How will the councils and the organization celebrate success?**

At the end of the first year, or the beginning of the next, plan a celebration of shared governance. Have all council chairs report on year-end goals and outcomes. Celebrate goals that were accomplished and outcomes that were improved because of council work. Another way to celebrate is with an annual report, newsletter, or announcement on the intranet of the outcomes, accomplishments, and improvements made by councils during the past year.

CHAPTER **THREE**
Shared Governance Processes

Once the structure is established (number of councils, council names, numbers of members, communication plans, and bylaws) you'll begin devising the processes necessary for the functioning of shared governance in your organization. Processes will include member selection, handling minutes, using the communication network, consensus decision making, and attending an annual shared governance retreat. In shared governance, the process is how you will function.

Responsibility, Authority, and Accountability (R+A+A)

Fundamental to the efficient functioning of staff councils is a clear understanding of each council's level and scope of responsibility, authority, and accountability (R+A+A). The language of R+A+A helps councils to build clearly articulated expectations, clear responsibility acceptance, and meaningful accountability checks into all their plans.[17]

---

17. Creative Health Care Management (2015); Koloroutis (2004); Manthey (2002, 2007); Wessel, Abelson, & Manthey (2017)

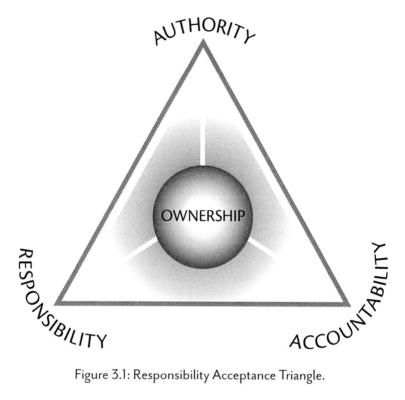

Figure 3.1: Responsibility Acceptance Triangle.

When responsibilities, authority, and systems of accountability are well-defined, a council is in the best position to own its decisions, as illustrated in Figure 3.1.

Responsibility

Responsibilities are one's duties and obligations and are listed in job descriptions, standards of performance, and scope of practice. In shared governance, general responsibilities will be found in bylaws. Specific responsibilities related to a project should be negotiated in a process that includes both allocation and acceptance of clearly articulated responsibilities. Just because responsibility has been given does not mean that it has been accepted.

The clear articulation of decision-making criteria is an essential step in transferring responsibility from leaders to a council, and it is one that is often overlooked. To be successful and make sound decisions, councils must know variables such as budget considerations, regulatory standards, vendor use, and scope of decision. These criteria must be shared early, clearly, and often. If councils are hearing "no" after they have made a decision, then decision-making criteria have not been clearly articulated. It is the responsibility of both leaders and council members to assure that they share or receive these criteria before decision making occurs.

Authority

Authority is "permission to act without permission." It is given to councils as their right to make decisions and act. Authority is only given after responsibility is accepted. Councils never have authority to make decisions without any guidelines. The extent of the authority must be clearly understood. Following are definitions of different levels of authority.[18]

Level 1

Authority to gather ideas and information and report to the rest of the team.

Level 2

Authority to gather ideas and information and make a recommendation for action.

Level 3

Authority to gather ideas and information, make a plan for action, and then pause together in order to communicate, clarify, and/or negotiate before taking action.

---

18. Creative Health Care Management (2015)

Permission should be sought only if the recommendation is beyond the scope of what the group is already authorized to do; otherwise, additional permission seeking is not necessary.

Level 4

Authority to act independently and inform others after taking action.

With rare exceptions, council authority should be at Level 3.

Accountability

Accountability is the review of actions and decisions and the evaluation of their effectiveness. Whenever possible, accountability is assigned to a specific individual to prevent the unproductive "everyone is responsible, so no one is responsible" scenario. With a culture of accountability—where we know who is responsible for what—the efforts of a council will be exponentially more effective.

Councils must take responsibility, have clarity about level of authority, and be accountable. One of the best ways for leaders to foster accountability is to *be* accountable and to *expect* accountability through clear structure and processes such as:

- Required reports

- Minute distribution timelines

- Quarterly review of progress towards goals

- Pre- and post-meeting communication methods

Steps for Effective Meetings

Before even putting together an agenda, an important prerequisite for effective meetings is establishing a common understanding of what constitutes a problem versus a reality. Sometimes councils get stuck when they are trying to address a reality as opposed to a problem. Clarity about the difference is important for success. There is no problem so difficult that it can't be solved. If it can't be solved, it's not a problem; it's a reality. We must accept realities and resolve the problems that come with them.

Distinguishing Problems from Realities

Here's an example of something that's a reality rather than a problem: An organization has a challenge related to adequate amounts of on-site parking for patients, visitors, and employees. There is no adjacent land to expand on-site parking, nor is there the ability to build an on-site multiple level parking structure. The fact that there is no ability to provide additional on-site parking options is an organizational reality.

However, there is also a problem in this example that can be addressed: Can the organization find alternative parking options? As they address this solvable problem, they can explore options such as reserving on-site parking for patients and visitors *only*, while finding off-site parking options with shuttle service for employees.

If the council determines that the issue they're discussing is a reality rather than a problem, they can adjust to the situation, try to minimize the negative impact, keep members focused on things that are within their control, and move on to subjects on which they can make a difference.

Agenda Planning

Planning an agenda is not as easy as it sounds. Often unit practice council agendas are created by the chair and/or co-chair.

Occasionally, especially at the start of shared governance, the unit, department, and/or service area leader may collaborate with the chair to prepare an agenda. When planning an agenda, think about the purpose and the goals of the council and follow them closely when selecting timely and relevant agenda items. Topics for council agendas can include:

- Issues related to practice and the practice environment

- New evidence and best practices

- Review of data including quality indicators, employee satisfaction, and patient satisfaction

- Reports from other councils

- Reports on follow-up assignments from previous meetings

- Items brought up in previous meetings that were held over for discussion at a later time, which are referred to as "parking lot" items

Agenda planning for the next meeting may start during the current meeting. As topics come up, or follow-up is needed, begin a list for the next meeting agenda. Make sure items are appropriate for the meeting. Allot a specific time for each agenda item. Allot enough time for each topic. If it is discovered that a topic requires more time, carry it over to the next agenda or create a task force or ad hoc committee to work on it. You may want to assign a different person to each agenda item to lead the discussion and review the decisions. During the meeting, items may come up that aren't on the agenda but need discussion at some point. Put those items in the parking lot and consider adding them to a future agenda.

To better manage your parking lot items (and prevent frustration for the people whose items get parked there), be sure those items are written down and visible to the group. Assign someone to monitor the list. Encourage and model individuals adding items to the parking lot on their own, or in other words "self-parking." Review parking lot items at the meeting's end, noting both the contributors and the content, and always follow up on those items. Do not let the parking lot turn into a cemetery.

Meeting Minutes

Meeting minutes are essential for documenting what happened during the meeting, including discussions, decisions, and exactly what took place. Meeting minutes are also valuable for people who could not attend. Meaningful minutes take a bit of work; devise a process for taking, reviewing, storing, and sharing meeting minutes.

Be sure minutes record dates, time, and attendance, as well as the names of people who brought up ideas. Write in complete sentences, spelling out abbreviations. Summarize what happened at the meeting and list all follow-up items and assignments.

Best practices include assigning a recorder, using a minutes template, and setting a deadline for completion. Establish a process for distributing and saving minutes, and have chairs review minutes as soon as possible after the meeting. Have members make additions and edits and/or approve the minutes. Email the final copy to members/units/departments, including upcoming agenda items. Then post them in all places your council has determined will make them visible to all who need access.

Principles of Effective Communication

Communication requires a sender and a receiver. Simply giving information is not communication. For communication to be effective, the sender must have credibility. Acknowledging others and using direct channels of communication are also essential. Responsibility for clarity resides with the sender, and concise language is best.

One sure way to block communication is through the use of conversation-stopping phrases, which have the effect of squelching new ideas and/or shutting people down.

These phrases may show up in council meetings. As a new idea emerges and momentum is building, a conversation-stopping phrase can come flying in, from seemingly out of nowhere. Members of shared governance councils, and especially chairs, need to be prepared to identify and turn around these phrases. A few examples are shown in Figure 3.2.

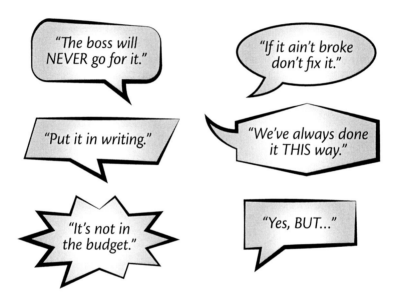

Figure 3.2: Conversation-Stopping Phrases

Turning Around Conversation-Stopping Phrases

It's best not to directly challenge the person. Instead, be ready for the negativity and kindly, with genuine curiosity, turn the phrase into something positive, as in the examples on the following page.

Yes, but...	Yes, and...
It'll never work...	Let's trial it. What could we learn if we fail?
We tried it last year...	What did we learn that could make it better?
It won't work...	How could we make *it*—or something with the same underlying intention—work?
It's just not *us*...	Let's look at what part of it is not us...

Communication via End-of-Meeting Summaries

End-of-meeting summaries provide a review for council members to recap major discussions and decisions from the meeting. Some issues from the meeting may not have been resolved and may not be ready to report to the staff. Other information must be distributed immediately in order to obtain feedback. A meeting summary is a great way to remind council members what to communicate to their colleagues, as well as a way to summarize assignments and create agenda items for the next meeting.

It works well to simply summarize key points of the meeting (e.g., top five take-aways), review assignments, list who is following up on which items, recap decisions made during the meeting, and list agenda items for next meeting.

Meeting Evaluations

Everyone wants to make sure the money spent on meeting time is money well spent, so it is helpful to conduct a brief evaluation at the end of each meeting. Ask members what went well, what they liked best about the meeting, and what could be improved. This sort of inquiry builds trust within the group while helping everyone to continually improve the process. Ideally this process is handled efficiently and becomes the group's preferred way to provide a sense of completion for each meeting.

Spreading the Message

Once the meeting is over, the work of communicating results begins. Taking the message to others is often a challenge. Ways to spread the message from council meetings include:

- Emails

- Bulletin boards

- Shared online resources

- Intranet

- One-on-one communication

- Communication networks

Keep in mind that the best communication is two-way, which enables the council member to get feedback and suggestions from others.

Using a Communication Network

Since council members are acting as representatives of their colleagues, it is critical that there be two-way communication between council members and colleagues. This council communication seeks colleague input and feedback on items the council is working on. It also offers a mechanism for buy-in of council developed plans. In a communication network, every council member is assigned specific people to inform. In addition to sharing information, a communication network is a great way to get feedback, answer questions, and learn about new issues that colleagues would like brought to the council. Figure 3.3 shows an example of a simple communication network.

COMMUNICATION NETWORK

Patti	Liz	Deb B.	Cristie L.	Kristy G.
Barb	Grace	Ezekiel	Jan M.	Wendy
Omar	Christy L.	Amanda	James	Kristy B.
Sue O.	Lisa	Michelle O.	Lauren	Vonette
Michelle S.	Judy G.	Theresa	Tiffany	
Abby	Terrie	Deb V.	Lezli	Jill H.
Harry	Nykkia	Terry G.	Carol D.	Lon
Melba	Dante	Travis	LeeAnn	Carol Z.
Sherree	Judy M.	Bansari	Jaime	Janice
Steph	Teng	Mavis	Toni	
Nicole W.	Tyschell	Jonelle	Tran	
Jill H.	Jessica T.	Inbong	Robin	
Carol B.	Ruth	Mary	Kacie	

Figure 3.3: Sample Communication Network

Decision Making

Shared governance councils are charged with making decisions for the greater good of the organization and for their unit or department. This principle is one that should be reinforced regularly, because it is easy for individual council members to begin making decisions from a personal lens as opposed to an organizational lens. In theory, there are several decision-making processes, including having the leader make the decision, using a "majority vote" process, making no decision at all, and reaching decisions by consensus.

While majority vote is likely the decision-making method that most people are familiar with, best practice in shared governance decision making is by consensus. In consensus decision making, the council members work together to find a mutually acceptable solution that all group members will support. It is not voting. It is not a show of hands. Consensus decision making is the judgment arrived at by most of those concerned; group solidarity in sentiment and belief; an in-general agreement and a collective opinion.[19] This does not mean the decision is everyone's first choice, but it does mean that everyone agrees to support the decision. Consensus decision making requires active listening, openness, honesty, dialogue, and emotional safety.

In our experience, the most effective consensus decision making is guided by these principles:

- Inclusiveness

- Flexibility

- Accountability

- Shared control

- Commitment to seeing implementations through to the end

The chair facilitates movement toward consensus using these principles. Group norms for consensus decision making should be established early and should receive special attention as the group becomes more comfortable with operationalizing the shared governance process. Group norms could include the following:

- Come to the discussion with an open mind.

- Describe your reasoning briefly so other people can understand.

- Avoid arguing for personal opinions.

- Avoid changing your mind just to reach agreement and/or avoid conflict.

- View differences of opinion as helpful.

---

19. "Consensus," *Merriam-Webster Online*

- Stick with the process and the topic.

- Make the decision for the greater good.

- Offer alternatives if you disagree with the plan.

- Share 100% of material and information needed to make the decision.

- Silence equals agreement.

As councils begin consensus decision making, it is important that they make one decision at a time. Asking a group to decide if they want item A or item B means requiring members to vote for one or the other. Asking if they want A, and why or why not, keeps the focus on one thing at a time.

Consensus is achieved when all people can state these three things:

1. I feel I have been heard.

2. I can live with the decision.

3. I will support the decision (no matter what my position was when we started).

It is important in the early stages of councils that time is taken to have each person state, out loud, all three statements. Council chairs must avoid asking, "Do we have consensus?" or asking for a show of hands for consensus, as this is just another version of voting. In a shared governance culture, solidarity surrounding decisions is critical. Council members also need to understand that speaking up and expressing their concerns or beliefs is crucial. Failure to speak up indicates to the group that the member is in agreement and will support the decision.

The ability to operationalize consensus decision making takes time, practice, and attention to process. Leaders must accept that councils that haven't been together very long will take longer to make their decisions. Leaders must be patient as their councils develop and mature.

The Council Facilitator Role

As councils develop, restructure, or attempt to move from a stalled position, a best practice to consider is using a facilitator. This role is not filled by the chair or co-chair or leadership sponsor of the council. The facilitator should be an individual who has no vested interest in the decision or outcome and no voice in consensus decision making. The facilitator contributes structure and process to interactions so the group is able to function effectively and make high-quality decisions. The facilitator's primary role is to pay attention to the process and ensure that it is followed. A skilled facilitator provides leadership without taking the reins and coaches others to assume responsibility. The facilitator is a helper whose goal is to support others as they achieve exceptional performance.

Think of facilitators as dealing in three domains; a facilitator could be a 1) content, 2) process, or 3) developmental facilitator. Of these three facilitator roles, only two are appropriate for shared governance.

A *content facilitator* leads the discussion and offers opinions with the intent to influence the decision or outcome. (Content facilitators are not appropriate for shared governance settings.) A *process facilitator* pays attention to group process, leaves content to the participants, and actively orchestrates discussion, while remaining neutral. The process facilitator's intent is to help the group move toward decisions and outcomes. *Developmental facilitators* are temporary process leaders who develop leadership skills in others, with the intent to work themselves out of a job.

A shared governance facilitator combines both the process facilitator and developmental facilitator roles. In early stages or when stalled, councils need an individual who will coach them on process and leadership. As the council matures and can manage their processes without external support, the facilitator moves into the background or leaves the group.

Facilitator Dos and Don'ts

Facilitators DO:

- Convey presence but not control
- Pay attention to process
- Foster a safe, productive environment
- Respect all participants and encourage mutual respect
- Educate about best practices, policies, and procedures
- Identify and clarify the interests and needs of the parties
- Model effective conversation and discussion patterns
- Protect each participant and help them save face
- Assist in collaborative problem solving
- Test the reality of what is proposed
- Assist in developing written statements and agreements
- Assist in implementation of agreements
- Foster leadership in others
- Teach and empower others to facilitate
- Point out when agreements are not kept

Facilitators DON'T:

- Control or run meetings

- Include themselves in decision making

- Violate confidential communications

- Assume anything

- Dictate agreements

- Impose their own values or preferences

- Make promises they cannot keep

- Enforce agreements

- Lose self-control

The toughest challenge as a facilitator is staying neutral.

When Might a Council Use a Facilitator?

The short answer is that councils may choose to engage a facilitator at any time to maximize success. One of the best opportunities to engage a facilitator is when councils are just starting out. Everyone is learning the structures and processes, and sometimes it is hard to remember what councils can and should be doing. The facilitator will help shepherd councils through the stages of team development and address the issues that arise with each stage. They will also ensure that councils adhere to the processes developed within the organization.

Another occasion to use a facilitator is when a council has stalled or is straying from the organizational structures and processes. The facilitator will ensure that these councils get focused and remain focused within the scope of their purpose and goals.

CHAPTER **FOUR**

Measuring What is Important and Maximizing Outcomes

Data must be the driver of all council work. The primary reason to collect data is to motivate people to improve practice. There was a time when patient care was not based on hard data. Caregivers knew what worked well by doing it over and over and getting the same results (most of the time). In the present health care environment, practice is data-driven.

Quality care means different things to different people. Think about the difference in what quality would mean to you, in any given situation, if you are a patient's family member, a physician, a pharmacist, a nurse, or an insurance company. A spouse of a patient wants the patient to be treated promptly and to be pain-free. The physician wants the patient's temperature measured and recorded accurately, in order to make the appropriate diagnosis. The pharmacist wants the provider to communicate medication orders clearly and accurately. The nurse wants the correct antibiotics delivered to start medication within a desired timeframe. The insurance company wants the PICC line placed in a timely manner so discharge will not be delayed. While everyone would be in general agreement about the importance of each of these activities, different people have reason to be focused on different aspects of quality care.

Quality Depends on Data

If the organization, department, or unit measures something, there should be clearly defined and measurable goals around the outcomes. Outcomes must be measured objectively and at regular intervals, and improvements must be quantifiable and sustained over time.

As a council decides what it will measure, look first at what is already being collected. What data is being reported and to whom is it being reported?

We collect data on a variety of quality indicators because it's the right thing to do, but also because it helps with reimbursement, quality awards, and compliance with regulatory standards. Nearly all health care organizations measure patient satisfaction (e.g., by using CAHPS surveys[20]), staff satisfaction, clinical outcomes, nurse sensitive outcomes, CORE measures, and more.

Data and Trust

Data represent reality. Occasionally, end users of the data may doubt the results. How many times have we heard, "There were not many surveys returned, so how can the data be accurate?" Or, after getting the results of an employee satisfaction survey, leaders have heard, "I don't know why they answered that way—they must not have understood the question." When such questions arise, the reliability of data must be assessed.

Reliability looks at how dependable a measure is under different conditions and situations. When November's patient satisfaction scores on a normally well-performing unit drop to

---

20. Consumer Assessment of Healthcare Providers and Systems, a program of the U.S. Department of Health and Human Services

the 50th percentile, we may interpret the data in a number of different ways. Depending on other circumstances (for example, a construction project that caused noise in the unit for the month in question), we might be able to say, "That was a bad month." One bad month does not constitute a crisis. Watching data over the long term and using trended data to create action plans is better than reacting to data on a month-to-month basis.

Reporting of data must be timely, or data may be doubted. If data is not seen as current, it is easier to attribute findings to environmental issues. Data that are months old also make it difficult to address performance issues and/or drill down to understand results in more detail.

Reporting must be planned at the outset, designed to reduce competition or embarrassment of low performers, allow for trending, be benchmarked, and be transparent about whether disclosure is full or partial.

Discipline-Specific Sensitive Indicators[21]

When it comes to deciding what data to collect, the simplest way to begin is to answer these two questions:

1. What outcomes do we always want to see in our unit or department?

2. What outcomes do we never want to see in our unit or department?

The answer to these questions can then be translated into discipline-specific sensitive indicators. Discipline-specific sensitive indicators are those items that:

- Reflect the impact of the care, treatment, or work done by people in that discipline

---

21. Indicators in this section have been adapted from American Nurses Association/ NDNQI (2010)

- Capture the care, treatment, or work most affected by the specific discipline

- Reflect structure, process, and outcomes of the care, treatment, or work of the discipline

- Contain measures of both patient-focused indicators and workforce-focused indicators

Patient-Focused and Workforce-Focused Indicators[22]

Clinical discipline-specific sensitive indicators can be divided into two types: patient-focused and workforce-focused. Nationally benchmarked, inpatient-focused nursing indicators that councils may choose to address include:

- Patient falls

- Patient falls with injury

- Hospital-acquired pressure ulcers

- Hospital-acquired infections

   » Ventilator-associated pneumonia (VAP)

   » Central line-associated bloodstream infections (CLABSI)

   » Catheter-associated urinary tract infections (CAUTI)

- Restraint use

- IV infiltrates

- Patient satisfaction

---

22. Indicators in this section have been adapted from American Nurses Association/NDNQI (2010)

Workforce-focused indicators that councils may choose to address include:

- Discipline-specific employee satisfaction

- Discipline-specific education

- Discipline-specific certifications

- HR-related

  » Skill mix

  » Discipline-specific hours per patient day

  » Discipline-specific turnover

- Safety-related

  » Needle sticks

  » Musculoskeletal injuries

  » Exposure to contagious diseases and/or hazardous substances

Workforce indicators should be tracked by people in every discipline.

Patient-Focused Indicators for Allied Health Professionals

Patient-focused indicators for allied health professionals are most often found in their professional practice standards. Examples include:

Pharmacy

- Wrong medication dispensed

- Medication order turnaround time

Physical Therapy

- Falls during therapy session

- Burns associated with heat treatment

Respiratory Therapy

- Hematoma post arterial blood gas (ABG) draw

- Missed treatments

- Treatments initiated within one hour of order

As targets are achieved and sustained for patient-focused indicators, the indicators will evolve and expand. For example, new indicators may be selected, or they may expand across the care continuum to the ambulatory and post-acute areas.

Key Factors about Discipline-Specific Indicators

Quality indicator data is most valuable when it is shared at the unit or department level. The data should also be benchmarked against comparable groups, including type and size of organization and unit or department. When these essential factors are considered, units and departments get a clearer picture of the value of their work and outcomes.

Shared Governance Councils as Data Managers

Shared governance councils, made up largely of clinical staff, provide a forum for data review and analysis and become owners of the data through the process of review, analysis, goal-setting, and action plans in response to the data. This supports the 2019 *ANCC Magnet Application Manual* statement, "Clinical nurses are involved in the review, action planning and evaluation of patient safety data at the unit level."[23] All nurse-sensitive indicators are patient safety data points.

Through presentation of the data and education, council members begin to understand the details of how data is

---

23. American Nurses Credentialing Center (2019), p. 42

submitted, displayed, and benchmarked. Sharing of data via shared governance structures ensures that data drives practice.

Challenges with Data Reporting

In many organizations there is a pervasive belief that data are only important to the quality department. It is even common in some health care cultures for reports to be shared only at the leadership level. As a result, staff members do not view the data as their own. Because of variations in reporting tools (such as calendar year versus fiscal year, varied subset scoring, and differing or unclear benchmarks), care must be taken to make reports easy to understand. That may mean that two reports are generated—one for use at the leadership level and one for use at the staff level.

Setting Goals

A goal is an intended or desired target with an identifiable end point. Goals are driven by data, align with the strategic priorities of the organization, and guide and direct the work of the councils. Depending on the council, the goals may also need to be aligned with nursing strategic priorities and/or unit goals.

Figure 4.1 shows some examples of an organization's strategic priorities and related council goals.

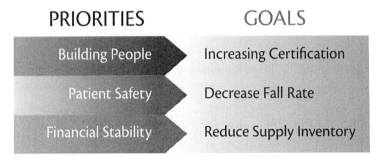

Figure 4.1: Creating Goals Based on Stated Priorities

Unit Council Goals

A great way to guide the work of the unit council is to set clear goals. Unit council goals are driven by data and focus on practice, the practice environment, performance improvement, and professional development. Every council in shared governance has goals, created at the beginning of every year or the end of the year for the upcoming year. They are discussed at a council meeting, so all members are aware of the goals, all members have input into goal development, and all members can create action plans to meet the goals.

Strategies for Successful Goal Setting

Create goals in SMART format: Be sure each goal is Specific, Measurable, Attainable, Relevant, and Timely.[24]

Smart goals energize the team, provide direction for the council, provide right-sized challenges for everyone involved, and help people think beyond the obvious. These benefits are summarized in Figure 4.2.

To set goals that are both inspiring and attainable, start small, both in number and scope. Focus on one to three goals, and tackle one goal at a time. Celebrate successes, no matter how small. Create solid, timely action plans, reviewing progress quarterly, or more often if needed. Assign tasks to various people, and make sure everyone has an idea of what achieving the goal will look like.

Councils set goals to provide direction and a sense of purpose. Not having goals is like sailing a ship across the ocean without a map. Goals keep the work focused and on track. Goal setting helps councils get organized, identify priorities, make important decisions, gain control, and create the council's destiny. One of the first items on the council's agenda should be goal setting.

---

24. Doran (1981)

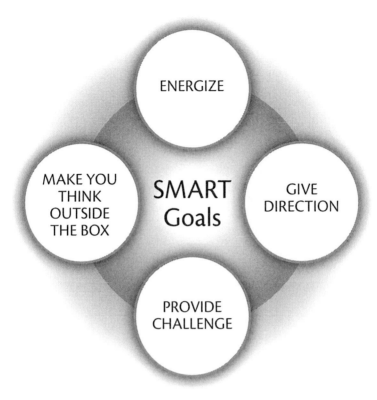

Figure 4.2: Positive Effects of Smart Goals

The five basic requirements for goal setting are:

1. A well-formed goal statement

2. An action plan

3. Motivation and commitment

4. A system of accountability

5. Frequent review and re-assessment

Goal Statement

Applying the SMART format for goal writing, make each goal statement specific (something desired), measurable, action-oriented, and realistic (within the council's control). Include a specific timeline for the goal, and be clear about how it can be achieved.

Goals formulated to achieve these standards are SMART goals. Again, SMART stands for specific, measurable, attainable, relevant, and timely.

Examples of SMART Goals include:

- Decrease the number of falls on unit ___ from (whatever it is now) to (desired amount—make it attainable) by the end of third quarter of [year].

- Increase the number of certified nurses on unit ___ by 5 nurses by the end of [year].

- Decrease the number of back injuries on unit ___ by ___% by year end.

- Decrease the medication turnaround time by ___% by end of Q3.

- Decrease the number of missed pulmonary treatments by ___% by the end of the year.

Action Plan Considerations

Consider what skills are needed to reach the goal as well as what information or knowledge must be gained to achieve it. Are there adequate resources to achieve the goal, or is additional assistance needed? What are potential obstacles to reaching the goal?

Motivation and Commitment

People will stay motivated if the goals are personal, feel consistent with the values of the group, and are realistic.

Accountability Partners

All council members should find accountability partners whose wisdom, knowledge, and character they respect. Make it someone who will accept no excuses for poor follow-through.

Frequent Review and Assessment

Engage in frequent review and assessment of the progress of the group. Make it part of a daily routine as well as a standing council agenda item. Frequent review will help you address unforeseen obstacles and make big decisions.

A Template for Goals for All Councils

Goal setting typically takes place annually as council members begin the year. Having a template for goals is a great way to keep track of progress toward goals, and document action plans throughout the year. The template should provide space for the name of the council, a purpose statement, the names of the council's members, a list of one to three goals, a space for action plans associated with the top goals, a space to indicate progress toward outcomes achieved, and a place to list accomplishments.

The template for goals can be very simple, as illustrated in Figure 4.3.

— **Annual Council Goal Report** —

Council Name: _____

Purpose Statement: _____

Member List: _____

Goal #1:

Action Plan(s)

1. _____

2. _____

3. _____

Year End Outcome:_____

Goal #2

Action Plan(s)

1. _____

2. _____

3. _____

Year End Outcome:_____

Goal #3

Action Plan(s)

1. _____

2. _____

3. _____

Year End Outcome:_____

Accomplishments: _____

Figure 4.3: Template for Annual Council Goal Report

Submit goals to the coordinating council (the council responsible for overseeing the creation and ongoing coordination of all councils) or on a shared space for council documents, such as the intranet, a shared online resource, or shared folder space.

At the end of the year or the beginning of the next year, gather the councils together for a "Report Out" celebration of shared governance. It is gratifying for staff and leaders to see the accomplishments from one year of council work. It's also a great opportunity for networking and for celebrating the successes of each of the councils.

CHAPTER **FIVE**

Evaluating the Effectiveness of Your Shared Governance Structure

At this point, you likely have many ideas to bring back to your organization, unit, or department. If shared governance is already in place, before implementing new structures and processes, consider doing a formal assessment that includes structure, process, and culture. If a formal assessment is not in the immediate future, there is still much you can do to assess the extent to which shared governance is alive and well in your organization or work area.

There are four kinds of assessments to employ to find out how well the councils are doing:

Formative Assessment

Informal, done in the moment; feedback is immediate

Summative Assessment

Formal, done at a predetermined time; feedback is delayed

Structure and Process Assessment

Formal, measures operationalization of structures and processes; feedback can be immediate or delayed

Outcome Assessment

Formal, measures what is different as a result of the
work being done; feedback can be immediate or delayed

Any shared governance assessment should include a periodic review of its structure, processes, and outcomes. *Structure* refers to the way the council is set up, including its charter and bylaws. *Process* refers to the actions or steps taken to achieve the council's goals. *Outcomes* refer to what is different as a result of the council's work.

It is important to know the difference between a structure and a process and to assess both, because a structure outlined in the charter and bylaws may not be what is actualized in the organization. For example, if the structure directs that people have term limits but the actual process is such that people stay as long as they like, the council should either revise the structure or follow a process that supports the original structure. If the structure directs that membership is formed by invitation but people have joined by other means, again, the council should either revise the structure or change the process.

Other considerations when conducting any type of shared governance assessment include timing of the assessment, how often assessments are deemed necessary, scope of assessments (all councils or select councils only), and who will complete the assessments (all members or select members only).

There are numerous options for conducting the assessment. Some organizations choose to design, conduct, and analyze their own assessment survey; others choose to purchase a pre-developed survey; while still others engage an external reviewer to do an on-site formative assessment or a combination of survey and on-site validation of survey results. Regardless of whether the organization purchases their survey or has it completed by an external reviewer, it is important to ensure that the survey is customized for the organization, is built on best practices of shared governance, and includes an analysis of results and a written report that includes suggestions for next steps.

Shared Governance Strategic Planning

High-functioning shared governance cultures engage in routine planning, typically on an annual basis, during a facilitated retreat that includes people from all levels of the organization. This planning meeting is used to determine what is working well, what is not working well, what the councils need to continue to do or stop doing, and what they need to do more of or less of. Some organizations complete a full SWOT analysis of their shared governance structure. Developed in the 1960s by business and management consultant Albert Humphrey, a SWOT is the process by which the group identifies their shared governance Strengths, Weaknesses, Opportunities, and Threats.[25]

Here is an example of a summary of a shared governance SWOT.

Strengths

Councils feature committed, hard-working long-term members.

Weaknesses

A culture of low accountability; acceptance of responsibility is absent.

Opportunities

Not all units or outpatient areas have councils.

Threats

Councils rush from one project to another without thoroughly evaluating or sustaining outcomes of prior projects.

---

25. Humphrey (2005)

Time should be taken at the retreat to review the current council structure and bylaws. Once these issues are addressed, the retreat can move on to developing the strategic plan. The shared governance strategic plan should be built on the organization's strategic plan as well as the division and department/unit strategic plans.

Enculturating Shared Governance: Individual Action Plan

If some semblance of shared governance is already happening in the organization, unit, or department, using a form such as the one shown in Figure 5.1 will encourage productive thinking about how well it's working and what needs to improve.

Consider the organization's assets and liabilities. Strengths are defined as structures and/or processes currently in place that are moving the organization toward the shared governance goal. Opportunities are defined as structures and/or processes that exist but need to be improved in some way. Gaps are defined as what is not there at all or is only minimally present. An example of an opportunity for improvement could be that shared governance bylaws are developed for some units but not for all units, whereas a gap could be that there is no orientation process for new council members or it is only conducted one time per year, while new members join councils throughout the entire year.

My organization's shared governance strengths are:
My organization's shared governance opportunities for improvement are:
My organization's shared governance gaps are:

Figure 5.1: Template for a Beginning Discussion about the
State of Shared Governance

The form in Figure 5.2 on the following page is designed to help individuals consider their own *personal* shared governance strengths, opportunities, and gaps. In this context, strengths are defined as talents, experience, and/or abilities that will help individuals be productive shared governance participants. Opportunities are defined as areas or skills people have and can improve upon. Gaps are defined as areas or skills they have never used or developed. An example of an opportunity for improvement could be a desire to hone one's listening skills, while a gap could be a lack of knowledge on how to use consensus in the decision-making process.

My personal shared governance strengths are:
My personal shared governance opportunities for improvement are:
My personal shared governance gaps are:

Figure 5.2: Template for Beginning a Discussion about an Individual's Personal Shared Governance Assessment

Using Felgen's I_2E_2 Methodology for Lasting Change to Improve Shared Governance

In the book I_2E_2: *Leading Lasting Change*,[26] Jayne Felgen provides an excellent resource for anyone planning organization-wide change. The I_2E_2 formula, visually depicted in Figure 5.3, begins with a clearly articulated shared vision and then invites readers to consider what changes are necessary to achieve the vision, focusing on Inspiration (I_1), Infrastructure (I_2), Education (E_1), and Evidence (E_2) (outcomes).

Felgen's methodology has been shown to work with smaller scale initiatives as well. What follows is an I_2E_2 plan to help organize a council's specific change effort.

---

26. Felgen (2007)

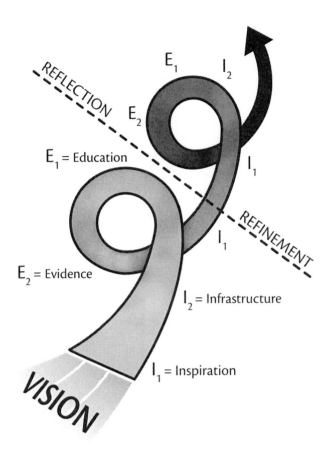

Figure 5.3: the I_2E_2 Model

Vision for Shared Governance

Describe the outcome intended, the way it will be experienced by staff and leaders. List all actions necessary to achieve the vision, including when they will be done and by whom.

Inspiration

How will the team inspire others and themselves to invest in shared governance? This would be the answer to "What's in it for me, my unit, my department, or my service line?"

Infrastructure

What must change in roles, responsibilities, procedures, systems, and norms in order to bring forth these ideas? What are the steps and timeframes? Who are the people responsible? Infrastructure includes council bylaws and charters.

Education

What education is needed to initiate and sustain shared governance?

Evidence

How will the team demonstrate or measure the implementation of this plan and the actual impact and outcomes?

Shared Governance Action Plan

Finally, we offer you a way to organize your action plans after reading this book. As you think together about what you will do to improve your organization, it's important to be clear about the full extent of your commitment. Use the template in Figure 5.4 to help you articulate and describe your commitment.

I commit to implementing these actions at my organization to strengthen shared governance.
ACTION 1:
Timeframe:
Challenges/Barriers:
Measure(s) of Success:
ACTION 2:
Timeframe:
Challenges/Barriers:
Measure(s) of Success:

Figure 5.4: Template for Shared Governance Action Plan

The Continual Improvement Mindset

The creation of a shared governance structure in your organization is not a "one and done" proposition. Instead, it will be assessed and improved continually. Know that the energy you direct toward improving shared governance in your unit, department, or organization will be some of the best energy you've ever spent. Every time you improve a shared governance process or structure, you'll be saving time, improving the output of the group, and, ultimately, improving the experience of patients, families, and everyone in your organization.

DEAR READER II
Our Commitment to You

This book has given you the basics of how to establish and/or improve your organization's shared governance structures and processes, but as you've probably guessed, this is one of those books that can only be brought to life through action. Lots and lots of purposeful action.

We have shared what we consider best practices as seen in organizations with strong shared governance cultures. However, the exact practices we've outlined are merely best practices—not requirements—and may simply provide a starting point for an evolution or adaptation that makes sense in your organization.

Remember, the structures and processes you set up today may not be what you are working with a few years from now. You can and should continually refine and improve your shared governance structures and processes.

Shared governance gives staff members and point-of-service people the responsibility, authority, and accountability for practice-related decisions. Ownership of outcomes and using data to inform and drive the work of the councils can help your organization improve such vital measures as employee engagement, patient satisfaction, and clinical outcomes.

We are fond of the Chinese proverb that states, "An owner in the business will not fight against it." Shared governance empowers each person closest to the work to think, act, and work like "an owner in the business."

Regardless of where you find yourself and your organization on the journey to enculturating shared governance, there is always opportunity to raise the bar. If you find yourself with additional questions or are seeing the need for consultation to establish or improve shared governance in your organization, we welcome your inquiries. We thrive when you thrive.

With admiration and gratitude,

Gen & Marky

REFERENCES

American Nurses Association. (2010). *Nursing: Scope and standards of practice* (2nd Ed.). Silver Springs, MD: Author.

American Nurses Credentialing Center. (2017). *The Magnet Recognition Program: 2019 application manual.* Washington, DC: American Nurses Credentialing Center.

Consensus. (n.d.) *Merriam-Webster Online.* Retrieved May 13, 2018, from https://www.merriam-webster.com/dictionary/consensus

Creative Health Care Management. (2015). *Leading an empowered organization.* Minneapolis, MN: Author.

Doran, G. T. (1981). There's a S.M.A.R.T. way to write management's goals and objectives. *Management Review, 70,* 35-36.

Felgen, J. (2007). *I2E2: Leading lasting change.* Minneapolis, MN: Creative Health Care Management.

Francis, D., & Young, D. (1979). *Improving work groups.* San Diego, California: University Associates.

Guanci, G. (2005). Destination Magnet: Charting a course to excellence. *Journal for Nurses in Staff Development, 21*(5), 227–235.

Guanci, G. (2007). Staff development story: Tips for a successful Magnet journey. *Journal for Nurses in Staff Development, 23*(2), 89–94.

Guanci, G. (2015). *Feel the pull: Creating a culture of nursing excellence* (3rd ed). Minneapolis, MN: Creative Health Care Management.

Hess, R. (2004). Organizational structures: For the people, by the people. *Online Journal of Nursing Issues, 9*(1).

Hierarchy [Def. 1]. (n.d.). *Merriam-Webster Online.* Retrieved July 20, 2012, from http://www.merriam-webster.com/dictionary/hierarchy

Humphrey, A. (December 2005). SWOT Analysis for Management Consulting. Retrieved from https://www.sri.com/sites/default/files/brochures/dec-05.pdf

Koloroutis, M. (Ed.) (2004). *Relationship-Based Care: A model for transforming practice.* Minneapolis, MN: Creative Health Care Management.

Manojlovich, M. (2007). Power and empowerment in nursing: Looking backward to inform the future. *The Online Journal of Issues in Nursing, 12*(1). Retrieved from http://www.nursingworld.org/MainMenuCategories/ANAMarketplace/ANAPeriodicals/OJIN/TableofContents/Volume122007/No1Jan07/LookingBackwardtoInformtheFuture.aspx

Manthey, M. (2002). *The practice of primary nursing* (2nd ed). Minneapolis, MN: Creative Health Care Management.

Manthey, M. (2007). Responsibility, authority and accountability. In Koloroutis, M., Felgen, J., Person, C., & Wessel, S. (Eds.), *Relationship-Based Care field guide: Visions, strategies, tools and exemplars for transforming practice* (pp. 486-488.) Minneapolis, MN: Creative Health Care Management.

McClure, M., & Hinshaw, A. S. (Eds.). (2002). *Magnet hospitals revisited: Attraction and retention of professional nurses.* Washington, DC: American Nurses Publishing.

Porter-O'Grady, T. (1992). *Implementing shared governance: Creating a professional organization.* St. Louis, MO: Mosby.

Porter-O'Grady, T. (2003). Researching shared governance: A futility of focus [Letter to the editor]. *Journal of Nursing Administration, 33,* 251-252.

Porter-O'Grady, T. (2009). *Interdisciplinary Shared Governance.* Sudbury, MA: Jones and Bartlett.

Swihart, D. & Hess, R. (2014). *Shared governance: A practical approach to transforming interprofessional healthcare,* (3rd ed.). Danvers, MA: HCPro.

Tuckman, B. W. (1965). Developmental sequence in small groups. *Psychological Bulletin, 63*(6), 384-399. http://dx.doi.org/10.1037/h0022100

Wessel, S., Abelson, D., & Manthey, M. (2017). Care delivery design that holds patients and families. In M. Koloroutis & D. Abelson (Eds.) *Advancing relationship-based cultures* (pp. 208-209). Minneapolis, MN: Creative Health Care Management.

ABOUT THE AUTHORS

GEN GUANCI, MEd, RN-BC, CCRN-K

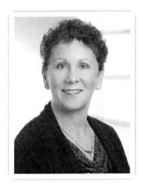

Gen Guanci brings more than 40 years of national and international nursing experience and skills to her role as consultant. Her expertise includes the development of strategies, structures, and processes to support all aspects of creating a culture of excellence, empowerment, and autonomy. She excels at helping organizations enculturate the voice of the clinical nurse though shared governance. Gen's passion is partnering with organizations on their successful initial or redesignation Magnet® journey. Gen was a participant in the 2013 inaugural ANCC Magnet Academy, which culminated in the attainment of ANCC's Magnet-related professional credential for consultants and health care professionals. Gen is the author of *Feel the Pull: Creating a Culture of Nursing Excellence,* and a contributing author of *Advancing Relationship-Based Cultures,* both published by Creative Health Care Management.

MARKY MEDEIROS, MSN, RN

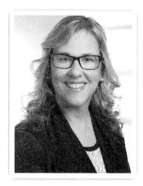

Bringing more than 30 years of experience to her consultant role, Marky Medeiros enjoys partnering with organizations committed to excellence in health care. Her dedicated work with creating and strengthening structures and processes in organizations can be seen in the areas of staff empowerment, leadership building, and shared governance, as well as coaching and mentoring as organizations create cultures of excellence. She has worked with organizations developing and evaluating professional practice models and is passionate about supporting clinical staff as they make the connection between professional practice and their daily work. Marky has experience in leading and partnering with organizations through all phases of successful Magnet® designation and redesignation. Marky is a contributing author of *Advancing Relationship-Based Cultures,* published by Creative Health Care Management.

ORDER FORM

1. Order Online at shop.chcm.com.
2. Call toll-free 800.728.7766 ext. 4 and use your Visa, Mastercard, Amex or Discover or a company purchase order.
3. Fax your order to: 952.854.1866.
4. Mail your order with pre-payment or company purchase order to:

    Creative Health Care Management
    6200 Baker Road, Suite 200
    Eden Prairie, MN 55346

    Attn: Resources Department

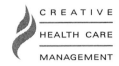

Product	Price	Quantity	Subtotal	TOTAL
B675—*Feel the Pull*	$24.95			
B690—*Shared Governance that Works*	$15.00			
B685—*Advancing Relationship-Based Cultures*	$34.95			
B560—*I_2E_2: Leading Lasting Change*	$24.95			
B682—*A Quick Guide to Relationship-Based Care*	$15.00			
Shipping Costs: Please call 800.728.7766 x4 for a shipping estimate.				
Order TOTAL				

Need more than one copy? We have quantity discounts available.

Quantity Discounts (Books Only)		
10–49 = 10% off	50–99 = 20% off	100 or more = 30% off

Payment Methods: ☐ Credit Card   ☐ Check   ☐ Purchase Order PO# _____

Credit Card	Number	Expiration	AVS (3 digits)
Visa / Mastercard / Amex / Discover	– – –	/	
Cardholder address (if different from below):	Signature:		

Customer Information	
Name:	
Title:	
Company:	
Address:	
City, State, Zip:	
Daytime Phone:	
Email:	

Satisfaction guarantee: If you are not satisfied with your purchase, simply return the products within 30 days for a full refund. For a free catalog of all our products, visit www.chcm.com or call 800.728.7766 ext. 4.

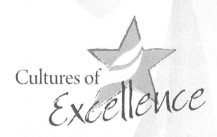

Cultures of Excellence

Organizations that partner with CHCM for comprehensive Magnet® journey support have a

100% Success Rate

**FOR JOURNEY SUPPORT
PLEASE CONTACT**

Gen Guanci
gguanci@chcm.com
or
Marky Medeiros
mmedeiros@chcm.com

800.728.7766

www.CHCM.com

Client Feedback:

"Creative Health Care Management helped us raise the bar and pushed our hospital to where we needed to be in order to gain Magnet designation."

"Our consultant was very honest and gave us "hard" news to help us accomplish our Magnet goal."

"CHCM has expansive knowledge and connections— the latest and greatest intel about what other hospitals are doing."

Creating a Culture of Excellence

Whether you are applying for a Magnet® or a Pathways to Excellence® designation, Creative Health Care Management can partner with you to ensure a successful journey.

Comprehensive Magnet® Journey Support: Full-spectrum support including document review and set-up, site visit preparation with mock site visits.

Readiness Assessment (Gap Analysis): Ground your planning and implementation with this comprehensive organizational assessment.

Re-designation Vulnerabilities Assessment: Discover where you are in relation to the current ANCC Magnet® requirements and uncover your vulnerabilities.

Shared Governace Support: Create or enhance the infrastructure of your shared governance.

Professional Practice Model Framework and Care Delivery System Design: Maximize staff engagement and ability to articulate how it drives practice. Increase the impact of your care delivery model with a framework that supports your organization's vision.

Professional Advancement Programs (Clinical Ladders): Foster advanced professional nursing performance, excellence in nursing practice, and professional growth. Create a framework that benefits the individual and the organization.

Peer Review and Feedback: Develop systems that enhance professional performance.

Data Management to Drive Practice: Leverage nurse-sensitive data that is meaningful to those who can change practice—staff at the bedside.

Magnet® Program Director (MPD) Coaching/Mentoring: We support and mentor MPDs regardless of their level of experience.

Magnet® Web-based Document Submission and Document Review Services: Easily access and edit your document anytime, anywhere with web-based document submission. Package includes comprehensive review of your sources of evidence.

THE JOURNEY TO BECOMING
AMERICA'S BEST HOSPITAL

CUTTING EDGE INNOVATION I

- Access anytime, any computer, anywhere

- Easy edits up until time of submission

- **Meets ANCC requirements** for electronic document submission

- Robust searchability allows appraisers and individuals in your organization to find what they need quickly

- Choose from design templates, customized with your company logo and colors

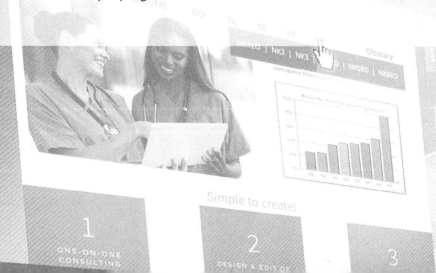